Traditional Healing and Beauty Properties of Citrus

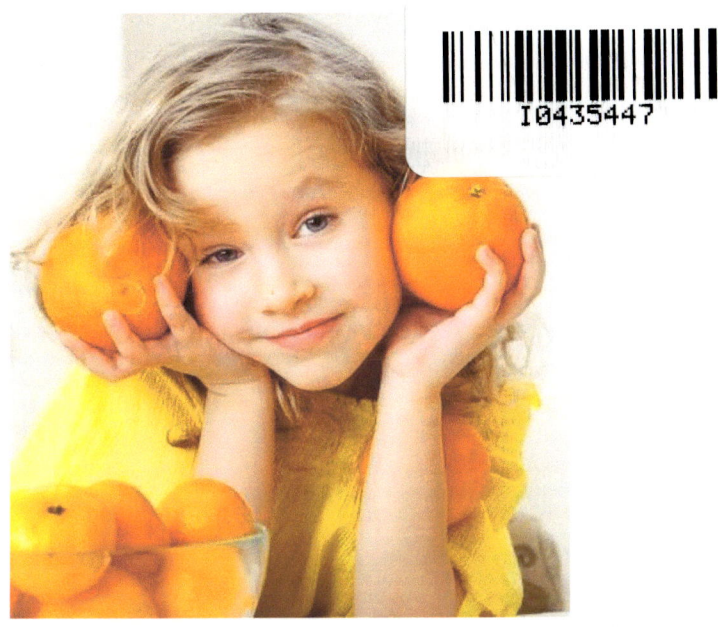

Oranges, lemons, limes, tangerines, and more...

Dueep Jyot Singh

Health Learning Series

Mendon Cottage Books

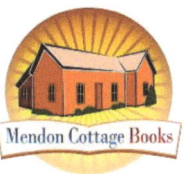

JD-Biz Publishing

Our books are available at

1. Amazon.com
2. Barnes and Noble
3. Itunes
4. Kobo
5. Smashwords
6. Google Play Books

Download Free Books!

http://MendonCottageBooks.com

Table of Contents

Introduction

I was just looking through some ancient medical treatises, translated into English and I was astonished at the number of times references were made to lemons, citrus fruits, oranges, tangerines, and kumquats to help heal and cure a number of diseases. These treatises were Asian in origin, Thai, Corian, Japanese, and Indian. Then I went to the Middle East and found that those ancients used lemon juice, in copious quantities in order to make up the basic foundation of a number of medicines, while their beauties used lemon juice in order to beautify themselves and keep themselves lovely.

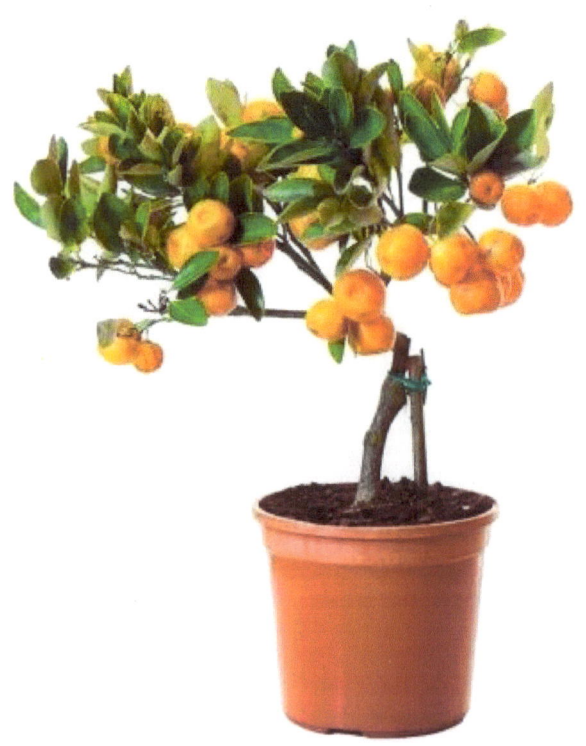

So this book is going to tell you all about the power of citrus fruits, in helping to keep you lovely, youthful looking, healthy, and best of all, with a product readily visible and available at hand.

Many of the citrus fruits are basically sun loving and that is the reason why when they began to be grown in Spain and Italy as well as sunny France, they were used just to keep the skin white. This was in the medieval times when health uses of lemons were not well known. However, in the late 17 century European sailors found out that after a long voyage, all they had to do was reach a sunny and tropical island, where there was plenty of lemongrass growing – this does not belong to the citrus family – or citrus fruit.

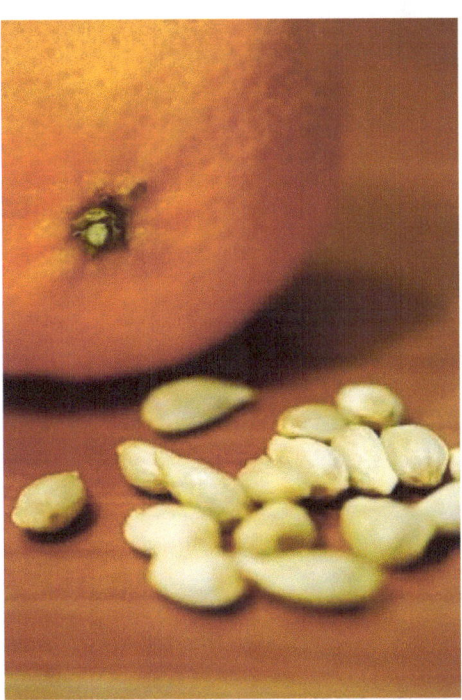

Columbus took orange seeds and saplings with him to the New World.

Their bad health was restored with plenty of orange and lemon juice drank. Their skin got back to a healthy look and their hair began to grow again. They also stopped suffering from scurvy and gum diseases. That was because of the large quantities of vitamin C in citrus fruit. So take full advantage of lemon – citrus limon, sweet orange – citrus sinensis – this originated in China, – bitter orange – citrus aurantium, tangerine – citrus reticulata , kumquats, and limes – citrus aurantifolia.

Many people think grapefruit to be a hybrid between oranges and some other citrus plants. They however happened to be a distinct species of plants in themselves. A trader named Capt. Shaddock brought it from Southeast Asia to Barbados and Jamaica in 1696. Because the weather was fine there, and it grew well and flourished, the sailors reaching Barbados from Europe were happy to have a good supply of vitamin rich grapefruit.

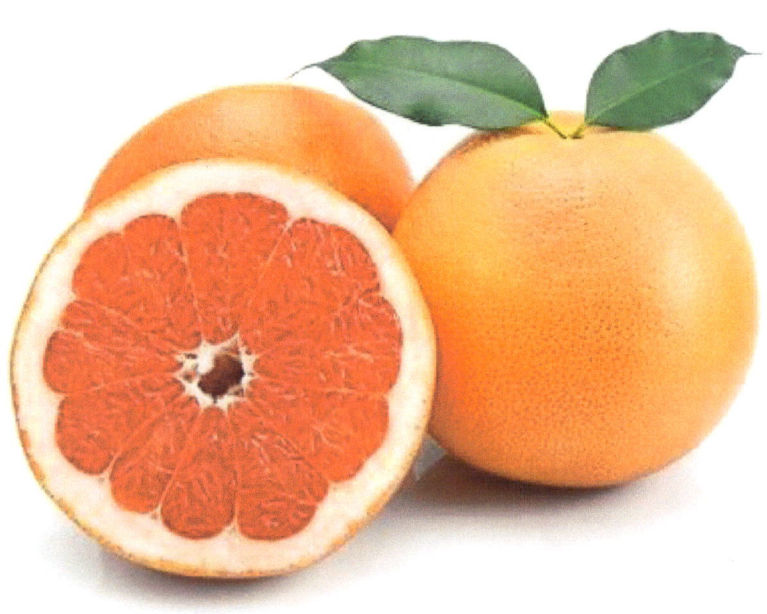

Incidentally, the word "limey" for a Britisher came from the addition of these lemons and limes to the daily grog ration of the British sailors. Blimey! As the cooks knew that the British stars were not going to eat the lemons on their own, the lemon juice was added to the rum to keep them healthy and to make sure that they did not suffer from scurvy. Just 1 ounce of lemon juice every day was enough to keep them healthy and fighting fit.

The first time I was introduced to a kumquat which is one of the smallest of the citrus family, I was surprised when I was told to pop it in my mouth rind and all! The rind was quite tasty and sweet. But oh my, the pulp, juicy and tart. Japan and China were the countries where kumquats first saw the light of day. That is the reason why you are going to find them in such abundance, accompanying Japanese and traditional dishes or in salad form.

Here is one hint – if you happen to be eating out, especially when the food is rich, Asian, oriental, greasy, spicy, or hot and you have a niggling worry that you are going to suffer from heartburn or indigestion, just go to the salad section. You are going to find a number of wedges of oranges there, which are going to be unpeeled. Just pick them up and add them to your plate.

Apart from the digestive benefits and the skin serving as a vermicide in your intestines, these oranges are well-known to prevent heart problems and ailments because they keep you healthy.

Limes and lemons originated in Asia millenniums ago and then they were taken to the other parts of the world by traders more than 5000 years ago. The ancient Romans knew all about lemons, which they got from the Mediterranean region, Spain, the Middle East, and from Asia.

Bitter oranges and sweet oranges are native to Japan, India, and China. The bitter orange was hardier than the sweet orange and it was the Moorish traders who brought these plants to parts of Europe, and the Mediterranean somewhere around the tenth century. Columbus took saplings as well as orange seeds with him to populate the newly discovered new worlds. He then planted them in Hispaniola.

Tangerines a very important part of Chinese herbal ancient medicine is called so because it was a variety of mandarin orange very popular in Tangiers. The flavor is delicate and sweet and apart from it being used extensively in Chinese cuisine, it is used to help in the curing of a number of ailments.

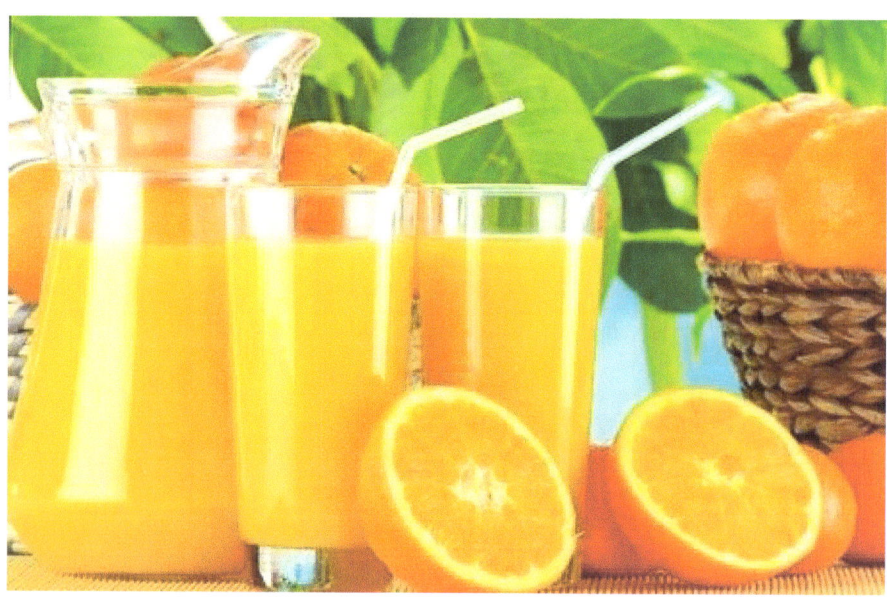

Citrus for Good Health And Beauty

Dental Problems

When I was a youngster, I never suffered from any dental problems because I knew the best remedy for bleeding gums and possible gingivitis. All I had to do was to peel a fresh lemon, turn it inside out, so that I could rub the white –zest portion on the bleeding gums for a number of minutes every day – either once or twice a day, depending on how serious the condition was. That got rid of any possible infections. I did not use the yellow portion on the gums, because that would mean my tender and bleeding gums stinging with lemon skin oil, not a good thing.

This would cure any potential disease on your gums, within a week.

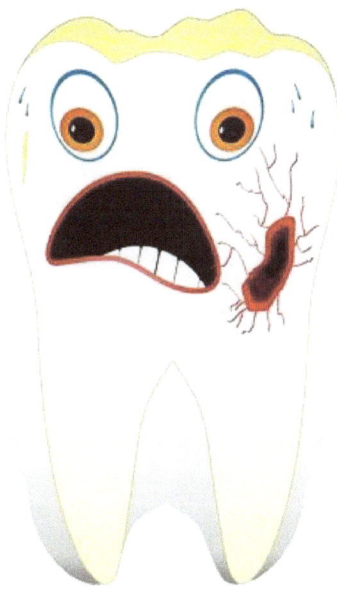

Here is the traditional lemon peel toothpowder which is used in many parts of the East, even today, in order to keep the mouth healthy and free of diseases.

Take 2 tablespoons full of dried orange or lemon rind. I would suggest that if you have a number of oranges and lemons, and the weather is sunny, just peel them and place them in the shade, – on your sunny porch – until they dry. Then powder them and keep them for future beauty preparations and for health preparations.

I once astonished one of the fresh juice stall owners in our locality, by asking him to keep some orange peels, tangerine peels, which he had peeled off the fruit, while juicing the pulp. He wanted to know what I would do with them. I told him that I was going to make some beauty preparations. He immediately wanted some of those natural beauty preparations for his family, while handing me lots and lots of fresh lemon, orange, and tangerine peels which I would then dry.

You are now going to add one tablespoonful of salt to that powdered orange and lemon rind, add a little bit of powdered cloves, ¼ teaspoon of bicarbonate of soda, and grind them all together. Use your middle finger to brush your teeth with this toothpowder in the initial stages, until your gums grow strong again and stop bleeding. Also, these are going to prevent your teeth from falling out, keep them strong and healthy, white and shiny.

In the same manner, if you have a lot of tartar deposit upon your teeth, just make up a mixture of lime, orange, and lemon juice and brush your teeth with this mixture, 2 or 3 times a week. This is going to bleach your teeth and keep them white. Also remember that if you have a habit of sucking lots of lemons, because you think that this is going to cure your colds, stop doing that.

Any sort of prolonged exposure to lots of acidic content present in the lemons are going to have a detrimental effect upon the calcium content of your teeth. So you may find yourself suffering from enamel deterioration.

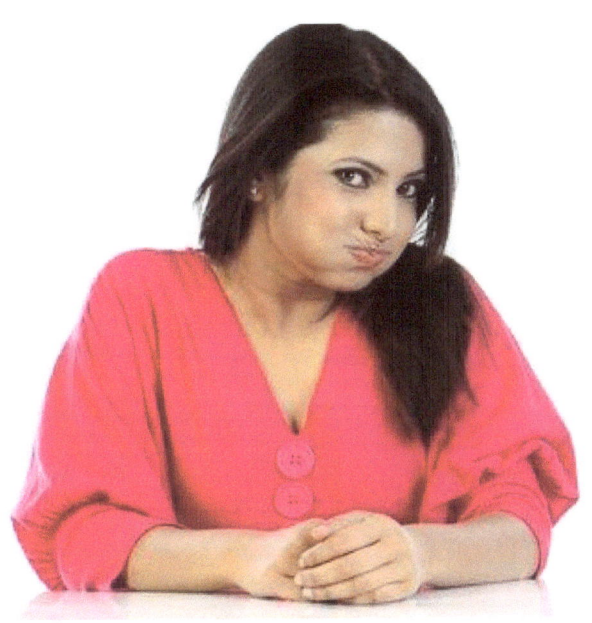

Lemon Juice for Toothaches

A mixture of orange juice and lemon juice is excellent to cure dental problems. You can also make a great gargle with a little bit of salt and lemon juice/orange juice in some hot water after brushing your teeth to get rid of the plaque.

The best natural cure for toothaches – apart from cloves is just to take some fresh lime juice and dip a wad of cotton in it. Now place it upon the aching tooth, and see the pain go away, in 5 minutes. This is the natural and timeworn remedy of getting rid of toothaches in times when one would not want to expose an ailing tooth to the ministrations of the quacks, witch doctors or barbers in medieval times.

Liver Cleanser/Gallstones Remover

This is an ancient Chinese remedy, and they use their own local oil, – sesame or any other oil – to make this up, but I am using 2 tablespoons full of olive oil, instead because it is available all over the world and easily.

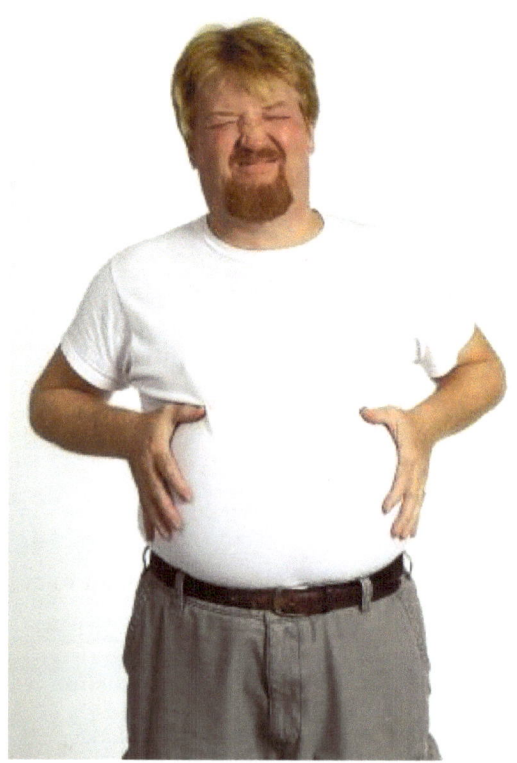

For this you will need freshly squeezed juice from half a lemon and freshly squeezed juice of half a grapefruit. To this, you are going to add 2

tablespoons full of olive oil. Try drinking this mixture, first thing in the morning for 5 days, and see the difference.

Alternatively, you can drink down two tablespoons full of olive oil, and then follow it up with half a cup of grapefruit juice. Naturopaths have been using this remedy to get rid of gallstones for centuries.

Fever Remedy

The ancient Chinese began their morning by drinking fresh orange juice and the juice of one lemon in warm water in order to detoxify their body as well as get rid of all the accumulated toxins build up.

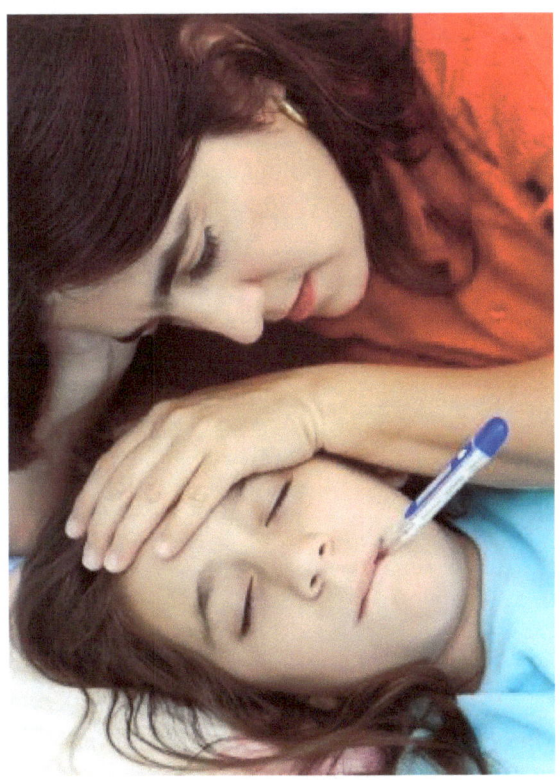

Also, even today, they make sure that anybody suffering from fever is going to be given lemon which is going to act as a cooling diuretic, lowering the high-temperature helping the body eliminate all the fever toxins and infection.

For this, you are going to take the juice of one lemon diluted in 2 1/2 cups of water. Add honey to taste. Give the patient this liquid to drink, so that he/she is not dehydrated. You can also make a cold compress made from the juice of one lemon in 5 cups of cold water to reduce the temperature and any surface heat or swelling in the body.

In ancient times, people suffering from fever were put on beds which were washed in lemon water and salt water to get rid of the infection. After that, a blanket bath – place a blanket over the patient, and wash his body with a solution of water and lemon juice – was given to him, to cleanse his body externally and get rid of the infections.

Lemon is a gastric antacid and alkalizing agent, even though it is sour to the taste which would make you think that it is thus automatically acidic in Constitution.

That means the excessive acidity in the body is going to be neutralized and any sort of sluggishness in the liver and the digestive system is going to be removed.

This is done by taking lemon juice in warm water first thing in the morning on an empty stomach.

Healthy Tangerine Tea

If you are suffering from body pain or just want to drink something which is going to relieve you of stress and body aches take some tangerine peels –

fresh or dried. Add the coarsely shredded or chopped peels from 3 tangerines, and bring them to the boil in 1 quart of water. After that allowed them to steep for an hour, and drink, mix this with one tablespoonful of honey after filtering. You may want to repeat this dose after 5 hours, especially if you are suffering from sore muscles from fever and flu and bones that are aching.

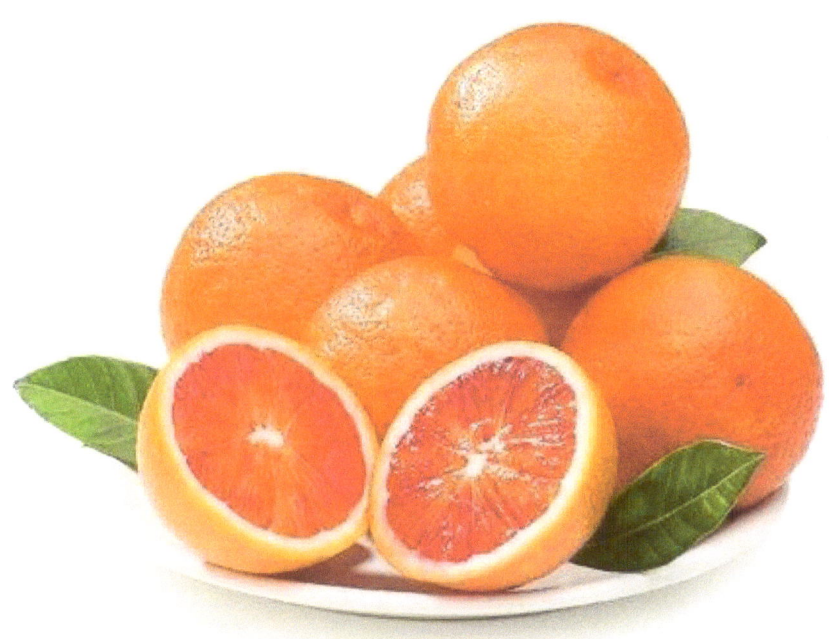

Let me tell you the healing agents which are being used here. The healing qualities of concentrated citrus essential oil in the boiling water, allowed to steep and then drunk with healing honey. What is not to like and take advantage?

In the same way, if you are suffering from problems of flatulence brought about by eating too many beans, just take the peel of 2 lemons and grate them in 2 cups of boiling water. Allow it to steep for half an hour. After that add the lemon juice and half a teaspoonful of honey and drink it down. No flatulence problems ever.

Natural Wrinkle Remover

Apart from its skin whitening qualities, a lemon is excellent for getting rid of rough hands and wrinkles, here is a remedy, which was told to me by an elderly woman who was in her eighties, but had a skin like she was in her forties. I could not believe it. The skin was flawless, and wrinkle free.

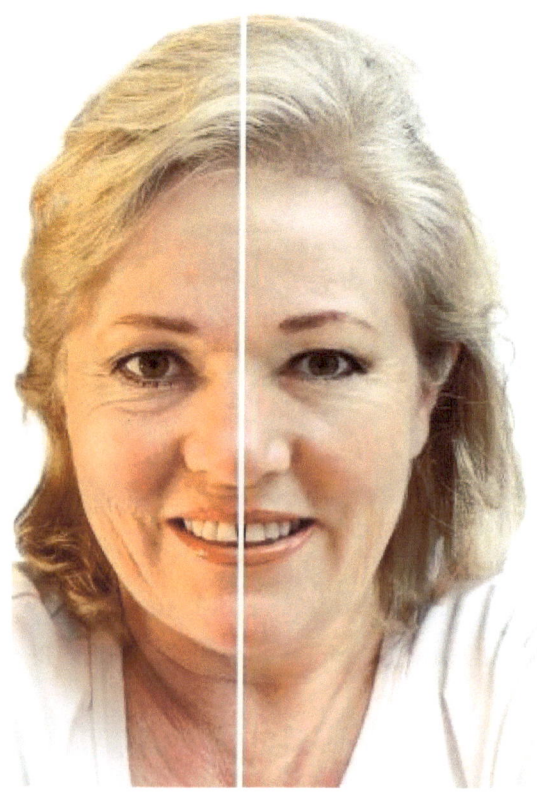

It was only when I saw her white hair that I knew that she was really old. You are going to take the juice of one lemon, add one tablespoonful of fresh milk cream, and one tablespoonful of lightly heated milk to that bowl. Make sure that the bowl is made up of wood or of earthenware.

Now add 2 slices of lemon to this mixture, cover with a little bit more of cream, mixed thoroughly and allow to steep for 3 hours.

This is the most powerful moisturizing anti-wrinkle cream available to mankind today. There are beauty salons asking thousands of dollars, for just one facial treatment using this solution massaged gently into the skin with the tips of 3 fingers, the middle, the ring and the little finger – these are the fingers, which are used in ancient massage system where you never use your first finger – the one used for admonishing, pointing, and all sorts of negative gestures! It is connected to a nerve, which does not allow the healing of the body, in ancient medicine.

Anyway, you are going to do the massaging for 2 minutes in a smooth rotating motion all over your face and the areas where you think that you can get wrinkles. Then leave it on until it dries.

After that, you are going to dip a washcloth in a mixture made up of ice cubes and lemon juice in which you have added a little bit of olive oil. Brrr, cold. I use almond oil, because I get it fresh in my area. Wash the lemon juice off and then splash your face with cold water. Do this morning and evening, and believe it or not, you are going to see a change in your skin, which is going to be lovely, rejuvenated and much, much younger looking within a couple of weeks. Try it out, I tell you it works.

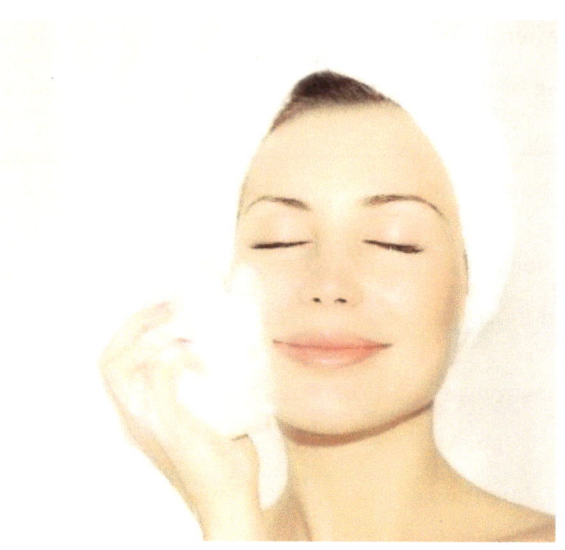

After all, the beauties of the East and also Egypt, Babylon, Persia, and other ancient civilizations have been using this cream on their faces for centuries, and that is why they were called witches by people visiting their country because they were so youthful looking, while their hair was all white.

So just imagine how much ignorance could be the basis of so much superstition, and a natural beauty remedy would have been considered the work of the devil because black magic was working here!

If you have very oily skin, you are going to use 3 – 4 slices of lemon and if the skin is very dry, you are going to use one slice of lemon. The lemon juice is to get rid of any blemish which is age-related. Remember to get the juice out fresh whenever you make up this solution.

I also asked this lady for her best hand softener, and she laughed and said, lemon dipped in warm milk and cream, along with the juice of half an orange. If you have too many blemishes on your hands, just take up some warm water, and put some lemon juice and a little bit of orange juice in it.

Dip your hands in that solution, and rub the solution thoroughly through your skin. Then allow the solution to remain on your skin for half an hour. Not only is this going to soften your skin, but it is also going to get rid of any sort of skin discoloration.

Do not go out in the sun after you have done a citric acid treatment. Citric acid is one of the important constituents of suntan lotions because it captures the sun and darkens your skin.

Here is another way in which you can get dramatic looking skin, really quickly. Just take 2 teaspoon full of Apple cider vinegar and 2 teaspoons full of hot water. Mix them together, and apply it on your skin to clean it and get rid of the dirt, dust, and grime.

Now apply fresh orange juice and lemon juice all over the skin until it is dry, and then wash with a moist cloth dipped in lemon juice and ice water.

Natural Lemon Skin Balm

Here is the natural skin balm which I make with 8 teaspoons full of rich sweet almond oil, four teaspoons full of fresh lemon juice, and 2 teaspoons full of clear honey. I used to add glycerin and Rosewater to the solution, in the summer to make sure that my skin was dust free. In the winter, it is just almond oil, lemon juice, and honey. I also added a little bit of fresh cucumber juice to this lotion in the summer because it was going to be kept in the fridge; amazingly effective and refreshing.

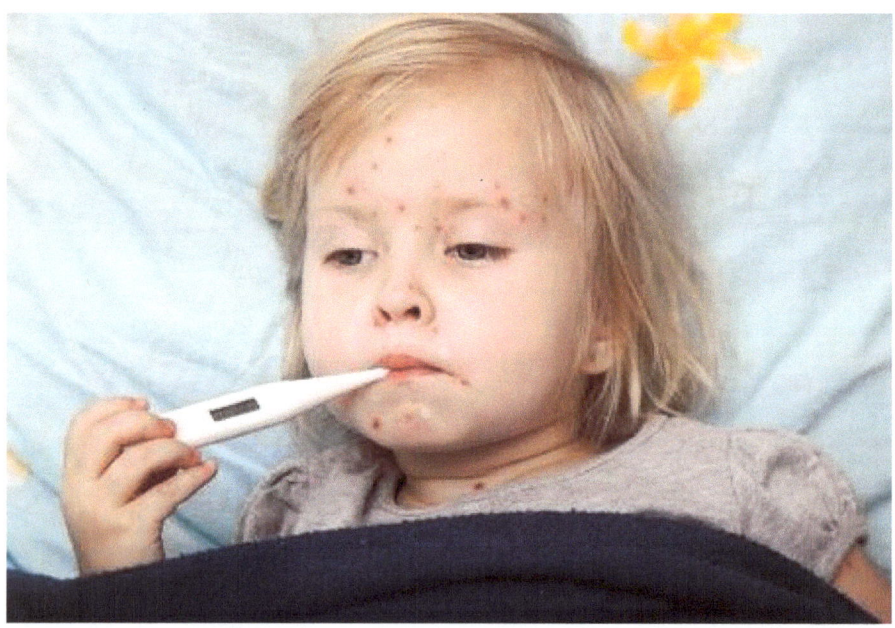

She needs plenty of lemon water with honey and when she is feeling better, the sport marks are going to be removed naturally and permanently with the lemon skin balm, leaving her as pretty as ever.

Make a lotion of this, by shaking well and is used by dipping a little bit of cotton in it, whenever you need to clean your skin and for moisturizing purposes. If you want a naturally perfumed body lotion, after your bath using amounts of water, with this lotion and apply all over your body. This is deliciously perfumed with the natural fragrance of the original products.

Remember that all the citrus fruits are rich in vitamin A, B, and C, as well as bioflavonoids.

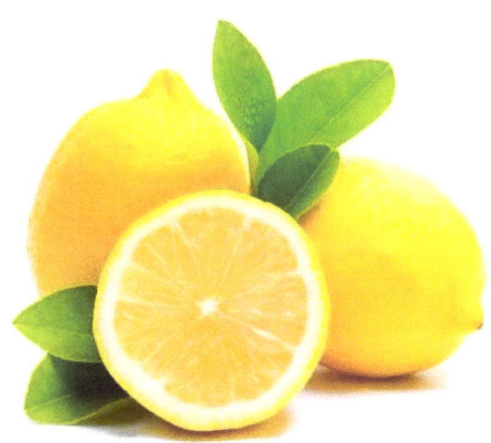

According to the ancient naturalists and those who believed in herbal magic, lemons were capable of attracting love, deepening friendships, purifying your home, and renewing youth!

Magical properties of lemon were harnessed by placing pieces of dried lemon in close proximity of whomever had experienced some negative state of energy or stale energy. You could also place dried lemon peel and lemon leaves in sachets, and place them on your cupboard.

There is the traditional purification process which is done when something bad has happened in your home, in the East, like a disease or something sad, by crushing fresh lemon leaves and allowing the oil to permeate the atmosphere. Then clean your whole house with these crushed lemon leaves in the water, which you are going to use to mop up the floor.

In the same manner, if you cannot find yourself sleeping well, due to stress and strain, just wrap up some lemon leaves after crushing them slightly in a muslin cloth and place them by the side of your pillow. This is going to get rid of any negative energy and help you to sleep well.

I found one of my friends making a traditional "love amulet" for a girl, who wanted to attract one particular boy, or even lasting love, in general. Girls loved those amulets! She just took some dried flowers of lemons and added some orange seeds to the mixture. After that she took a piece of lemon peel and orange peel and squirted the essential oil over the mixture.

This was then folded up carefully in a small silver amulet cover and handed over to the person who wanted this amulet, which she was going to wear around her neck! I wonder about whether it was just autosuggestion, or just the lady had a belief in herself that she was attractive and she soon found her partner and her much wanted happily ever after.

No wonder the wise old ladies of the East and of the Orient were considered to be well versed in love – lotions and potions!

Grapefruit Heartburn Cure

Here is a remedy, of which not many people know. For this, you are going to take a ripe grapefruit and remove all the colored outer portion. You are left with some threads and some white portion. This white portion is the most important portion for getting rid of heartburn and stomach problems, including indigestion.

Spread it all on a white cotton cloth and place it in the shade, until it gets dry and crinkled looking. You can either grate them before hand before you dry them, or let them remain in the broken up condition, they were originally when you peeled them.

Whenever you have a feeling of heartburn or even an upset stomach, just take ¾ teaspoons full of this mixture and suck until you feel your stomach settling.

Curing Diverticulitis and Diarrhea

Diverticulitis is the inflammation of the colon where you are going to have problems, discomfort, and pain while eliminating waste. This can be prevented and cured by eating lots of oranges. Also, if you are suffering from diarrhea, just the juice of half a lemon in very hot water and drink it down. Apart from it being a restorative of essential minerals and salts in children and babies suffering from diarrhea, the elderly can also benefit from this treatment.

Lemons for Headaches And Migraines

If you suffer from stress, headaches, tension headaches, or chronic migraines, you may want to try this natural remedy used by women in Indonesia.

The moment they feel a tension headache coming on, they just go and wash some utensils or clothes, by hand. Incidentally, the way of washing clothes in Asia traditionally is to rub lots of soap into them, allowing the soap suds to foam, and then beating and rubbing the clothes placed on the floor with their hands and also beating them on rocks!

Not only does this get rid of all the grime but I would not be surprised if it got rid of all the stress and tension accumulated in your body because you are pounding something until it cries for mercy!

Nevertheless, scientists have an explanation for this washing utensils in the hot soapy water thing, in which they have put the juice of one lemon or washing the clothes in hot soapy water with lemon added.

Apart from your hands working, the lemon water is capable of getting all the blood accumulated in the head region and causing the tension headache or migraine to the hands because muscular exercise is being done there. This also reduces the swelling of the muscular tissue in the head region, and gets rid of the headache.

If you are suffering from a really severe chronic migraine, which does not seem to go away, stand up straight, upright, and barefoot in a large enough foot bowl in which you have put hot water with the juice of one lemon added. This is going to get rid of the headache with the tension going out straight throughout your upright body out of your feet into the lemon water and the hot water, soothing the pressure points at the base of your feet with lemon.

If you do not want to go and stand before the sink washing utensils you can try out another remedy to cure a headache.

For this you are going to take a lemon skin and place the white portion on a piece of cotton handkerchief. Now you are going to take the yellow portion and apply it to your forehead, through the handkerchief all over the aching region. When you feel a burning sensation coming on, due to the essential oils burning into your skin, which means your headache is going to go away. No more migraines.

Guaranteed success.

Incidentally, I was reading Thor Heyerdahl's book *Fatu Hiva* in which he suggests a really excellent way in which you can get rid of the pain from bee stings, Wasp and centipede stings and bites, as well as mosquito bites and stings.

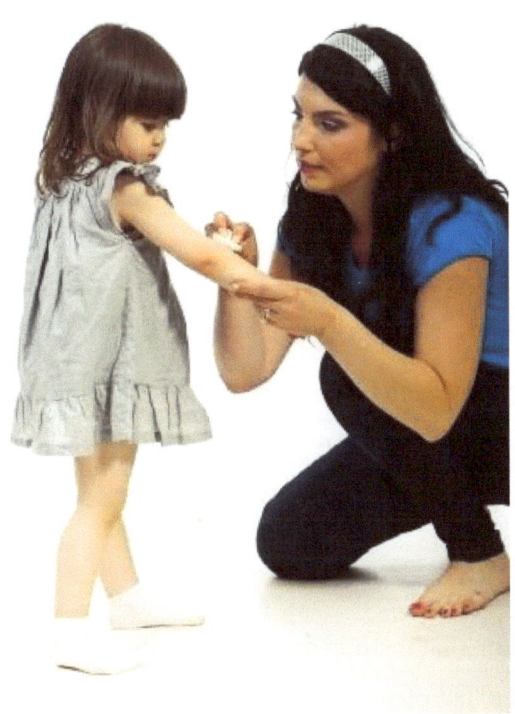

Just put some fresh lemon juice over that affected area and within 5 minutes, you are not going to feel any pain, irritation, or sting. Well, I would not be surprised that he found this remedy when he was sailing *Kon Tiki*, with all its insect life, sharing his boat on the high seas.

In the same way, here are the ancient magic supposedly related with the orange – Citrus auranthium – an orange plant growing in your house encouraged prosperity, attracted love, and dispelled negativity!

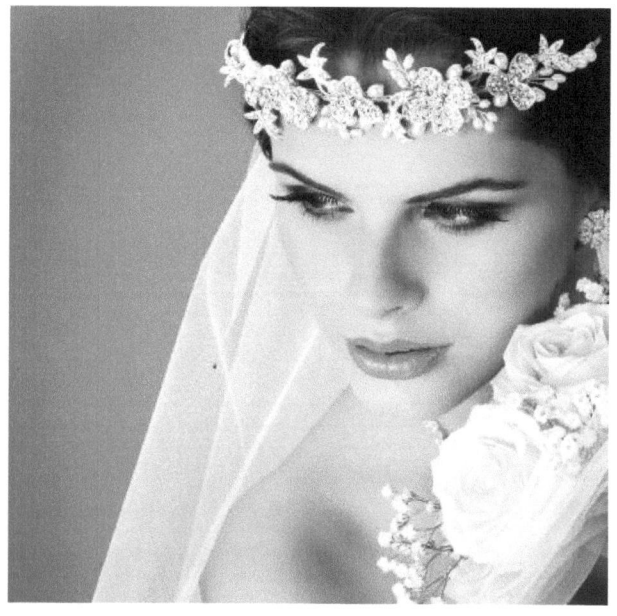

In many traditional marriage ceremonies, the bride is going to have orange blossom either in her bridal bouquet or in her floral decorations, as well as on the altar.

Incidentally, I think that there in something in this, because all the gardens which I had which had plenty of oranges and lemons growing there had me very happy, personally, financially secure and with not much family tension! But then magic related to plants may be mumbo-jumbo with no scientific basis but the feeling has come down through ancient times, where the belief was that citrus auranthium would show you how to find true prosperity and true happiness!

Remember I told you about orange seeds in the amulet? That is because the belief was that these orange seeds would flourish only in lands where there was plenty of sun and water, and that is why they needed plenty of nurturing.

In ancient Chinese as well as oriental/Asian and even some Middle Eastern stories where a fairy princess would live in an orange given to the hero by a good witch, she always asked for water, the moment the orange was cut. In many stories, the hero was given 3 lemons because being quite foolish, he would cut 2 lemons and have no water at hand, and the fairies would escape.

But then being the hero he would have a pitcher full of water ready at hand for the third fairy princess who would of course be the most beautiful one of them all, and when she asked for water, he would give her lots of water and she would stay with him forever and ever.

So that is the idea about love being cherished and nourished when care is taken, in the case of oranges and lots of water given too. There seems to be an analogy somewhere here, in matters of relationships and in matters of growing plants.

Do you know the reason why orange blossoms are part and parcel of so many weddings in so many cultures all over the world, including a white wedding with orange blossom? You may not know that this comes down from ancient times when pagan weddings were always held in orange orchards with the orange seeds symbolizing happiness, love, and fertility and the orange blossoms getting rid of all the evil, negativity, and a new start to a true and loving relationship.

Also, none of these weddings would have been complete without a number of bowls filled with oranges placed on the altar during the marriage ceremony and then the fruit distributed among all the guests so that they could also partake of the joy, happiness, and the blessings of the ancient Gods and ancestors on such a happy occasion.

Here is one of those old poems,

My love/the orange blossom/nestling in my bosom/rains up on me blessings / my heart held in her dainty white hands/my fragrant white orange blossom.

So there is some symbolism going back to ancient civilizations regarding the orange blossom. As far as I think, this is because the tree blossoms and bears fruit at the same time. Also, the flower is so sweet smelling and the fruit so orange, happy looking and delicious when ripe!

And if you get scratched by the thorns, while you are plucking lemons, just rub a little bit of orange rind on that scratched area, and it is going to heal without any infection!

Traditional Lemon Garlic Honey

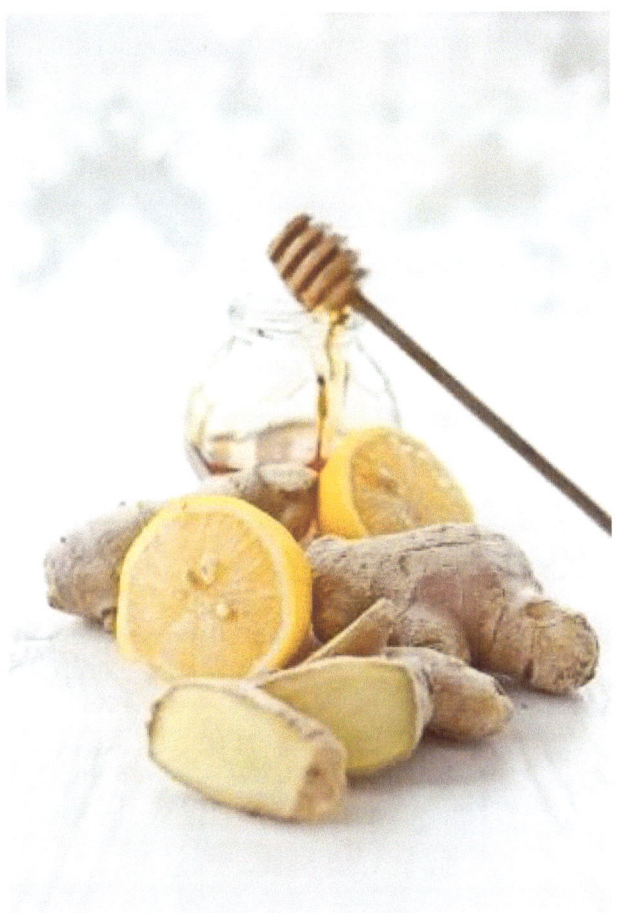

The combination of ginger, lemon, and honey has been known since ancient times to help combat chest infections, respiratory problems, sore throat, coughs, and colds in the winter. Just add juice of half the lemon, to a little bit of grated ginger, with one tablespoonful of honey. Drink after every 2 hours until totally cured.

The honey garlic lemon tonic is an ancient strengthening restorative, a preventative tonic, and also a remedy of treatment which has been used for ages to help cure people of ailments.

For this, when you are using it as a preventative or as a tonic, you are going to take half a teaspoonful daily.

When you are using it as a curative for a number of ailments, – you can consider this to be a basic multipurpose cure-all for any sort of non-chronic ailments – coughs colds, fevers, getting rid of toxins, curing your lungs, curing yourself of respiratory problems, you are going to heal yourself with this very powerful tonic. As a remedy, half teaspoon, 3 times a day, or 6 times, if you are healing a really acute chronic condition.

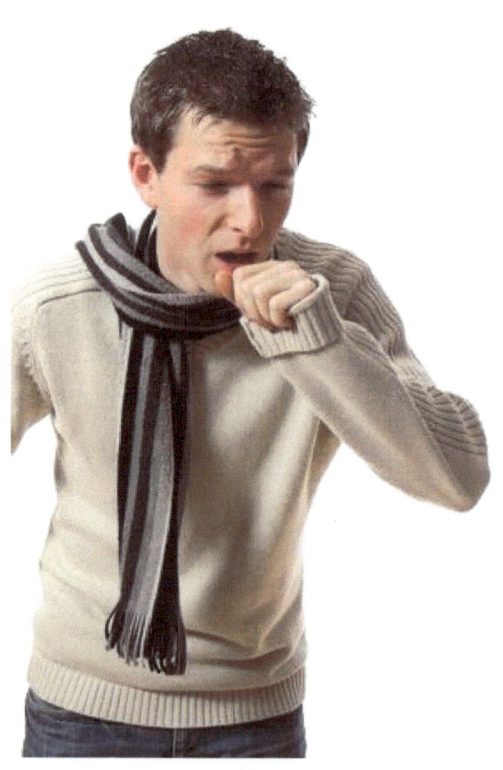

That is because the honey is a natural antibiotic and antiseptic and so is the garlic and the lemon.

Take 2 whole heads of garlic – fat, juicy cloves, preferably organic garlic. In our neck of woods, where everybody is rather lazy and cannot be bothered to peel garlic from the heads, the local market has another idea. They break the garlic off the heads and sell it at about 5% more than the ones still there in the heads. Somehow we buy the more expensive and already de – headed garlic, though, because it is loose, we use larger quantities of it in our cooking!

Nevertheless, you are going to take the dosage either directly or add to lemon and water, or even milk.

However, you may find yourself exhaling garlic! That is because the lungs are being disinfected during the exhaling process and the scent of garlic on your breath means that it is efficacious and is doing its work.

You can also use this honey as a disinfectant directly on your skin for scratches, bites, and wounds.

You are going to dilute one teaspoonful in 2 cups of water as an antiseptic skin lotion. You can rub garlic honey on the soles of little childrens' feet to keep them healthy.

First peel the garlic heads, slice off the bases of the cloves and crush them in a garlic press. Put the crushed garlic in a pestle and mortar and pound them until they become semitransparent. Crushing is going to release the active compounds already present in the garlic. Keep adding some drops of lemon juice, when you are doing the crushing.

Now add 2 tablespoons full of honey to this garlic and continue the crushing process. Alternate with honey and lemon juice until the garlic is totally transparent. Now add the remaining honey and mix properly.

Now you are going to take a glass bottle and put 2 small slices of lemon – properly washed before hand – into the bottle before you pour this garlic honey into the bottle. This is going to keep indefinitely.

Incidentally, I've tried this on my family, especially when they were suffering from fever and because it is digested properly and easily, this soon restored them to good health, especially my 84-year-old father in the winter.

So this is extremely health giving for babies, children, and the elderly. You can drink this as a tonic to keep healthy and youthful looking. You can give it to your children and grandchildren so that they have a really strong immune system, clear skin, healthy bones, and muscular growth.

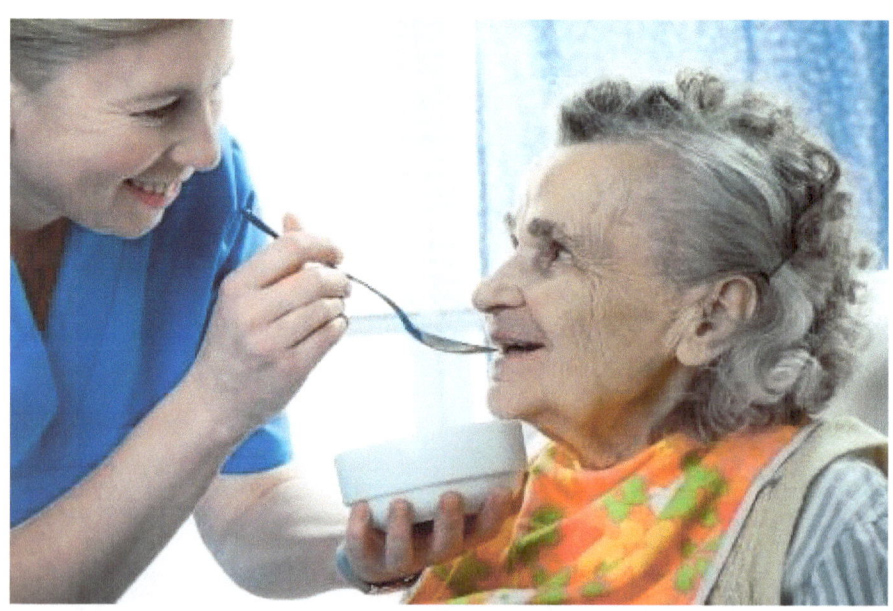

Conclusion

This book has given you plenty of information about the healing powers as well as the beauty and restorative powers of citrus fruits and plants. All of the remedies given here have been time-tested.

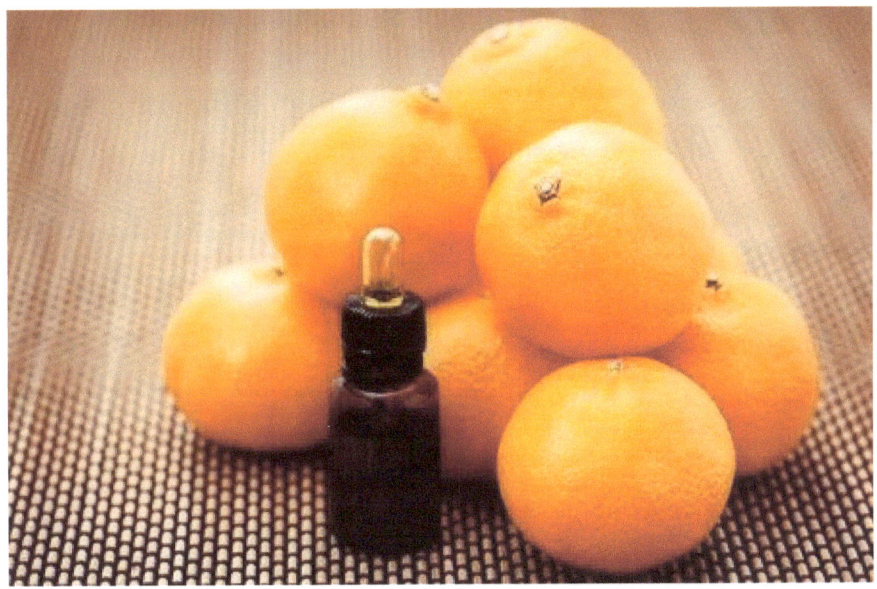

Remember the orange powder of which I was talking some time ago, made from the peel borrowed from a fresh fruit juice vendor? That is the best skin cleansing scrub you can get anywhere in the world.

Make sure it is properly powdered, before you add a little bit of honey to it. Now apply it as a paste all over your face and start rubbing your skin slowly in circular motions. This is going to get rid of any grime and also the dead cells on the surface of the body.

When I do not want to use it as a scrub, I use it as a facemask with honey, milk, and orange peel paste. I add a little of sandalwood powder, if it is a special occasion and I want my skin to smelled fragrant naturally. And then I apply this paste all over my skin, and allow it to dry. I then rub it off with warm water, so that I get a beautifully moisturized sweet smelling good-looking skin, without any resort to any other chemical-based creams, powders, measuring lotions, and potions ever again.

And at night, if I think that my skin needs a little bit more whitening, because I have been out in the sun, and it has caught suntan, I am going to wash my face with hot water – no soap, I have never used soap – and then apply lemon juice all over that suntan, and then good night.

Tomorrow morning I am going to scrub my face with warm water in the shower, and apply the lemon body lotion, given above, if I do not intend to go out and so I can sit bleaching out comfortably in the house itself.

But if I am going out, I am going to protect the skin with a lotion of honey and water and a covering. When I can manage it, I am going to get rid of the dust and grime with a bottle in my purse in which I have made a lotion of cucumber and Rosewater. The Rosewater keeps my skin hydrated, the cucumber cleans it and keeps it looking young and fresh.

So now that you know more about the traditional healing and beauty treatments which you can get from citrus fruit, you can add them to your daily shopping list right now.

Never peel an orange before eating it, unless of course you are using it as decoration. If you are eating it just like that, wash it thoroughly to get rid of all the accumulated dust and pesticides, and then chomp along with the skin. The skin has essential oils with lots of precious antifungal properties. The underneath portion of the skin also has essential nutrients which are really healthy and which are going to have enough fiber to keep your system moving properly, especially your digestion.

Live Long and Prosper!

Author Bio

Dueep Jyot Singh is a Management and IT Professional who managed to gather Postgraduate qualifications in Management and English and Degrees in Science, French and Education while pursuing different enjoyable career options like being an hospital administrator, IT,SEO and HRD Database Manager/ trainer, movie , radio and TV scriptwriter, theatre artiste and public speaker, lecturer in French, Marketing and Advertising, ex-Editor of Hearts On Fire (now known as Solstice) Books Missouri USA, advice columnist and cartoonist, publisher and Aviation School trainer, ex-moderator on Medico.in, banker, student councilor ,travelogue writer … among other things!

One fine morning, she decided that she had enough of killing herself by Degrees and went back to her first love -- writing. It's more enjoyable! She already has 48 published academic and 14 fiction- in- different- genre books under her belt.

When she is not designing websites or making Graphic design illustrations for clients , she is browsing through old bookshops hunting for treasures, of which she has an enviable collection – including R.L. Stevenson, O.Henry, Dornford Yates, Maurice Walsh, De Maupassant, Victor Hugo, Sapper, C.N. Williamson, "Bartimeus" and the crown of her collection- Dickens "The Old Curiosity Shop," and "Martin Chuzzlewit" and so on… Just call her "Renaissance Woman" - collecting herbal remedies, acting like Universal Helping Hand/Agony Aunt, or escaping to her dear mountains for a bit of exploring, collecting herbs and plants, and trekking.

Check out some of the other JD-Biz Publishing books

Gardening Series on Amazon

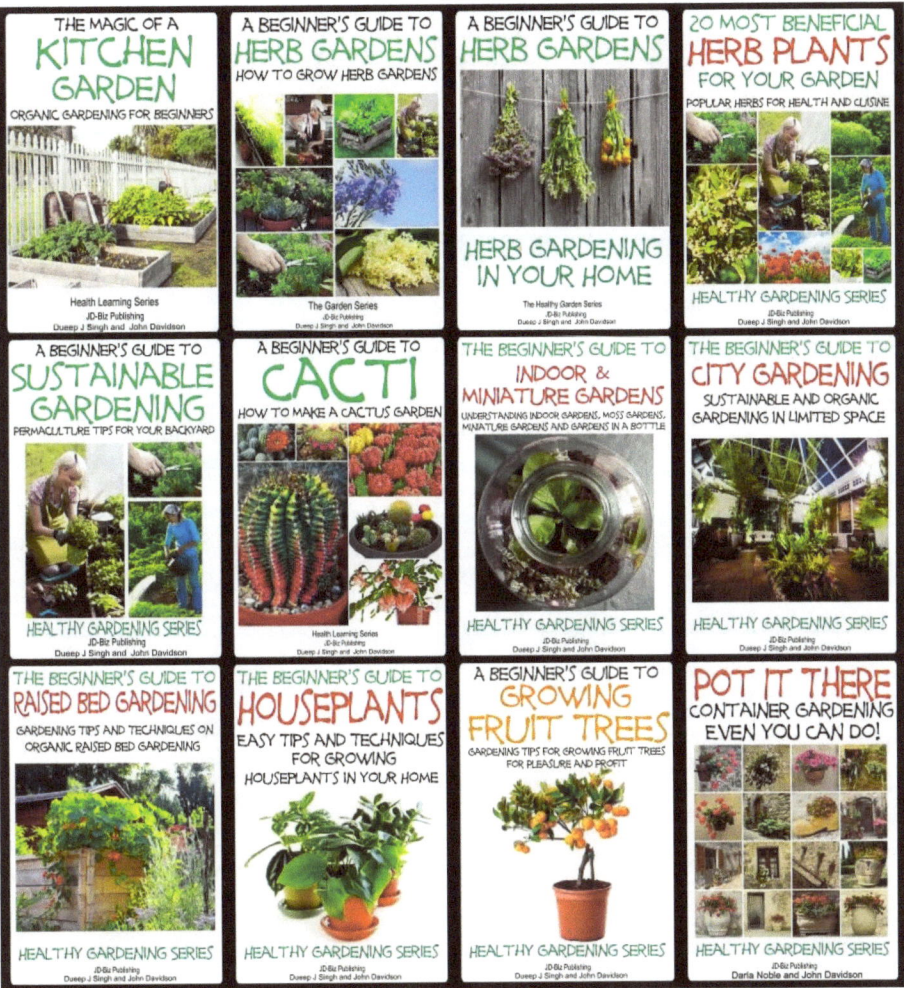

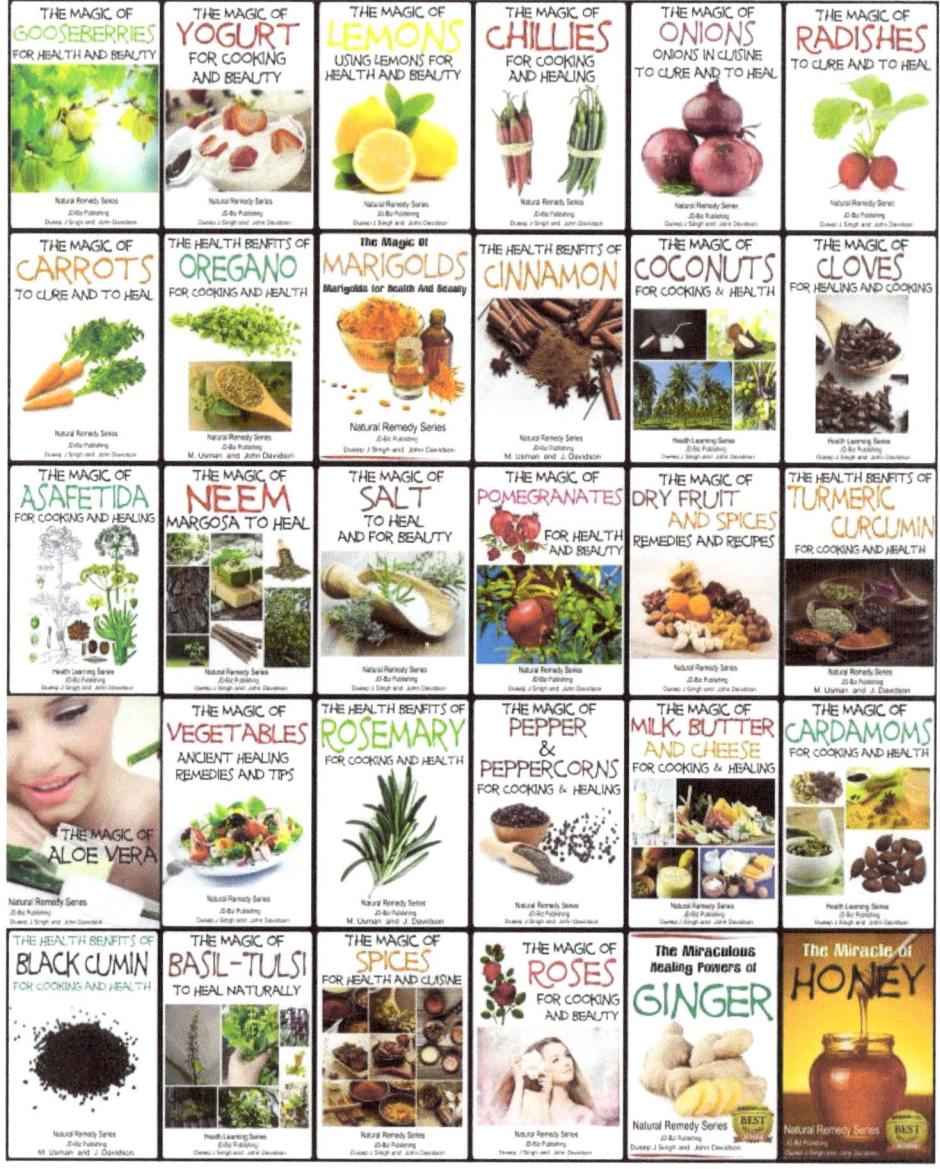

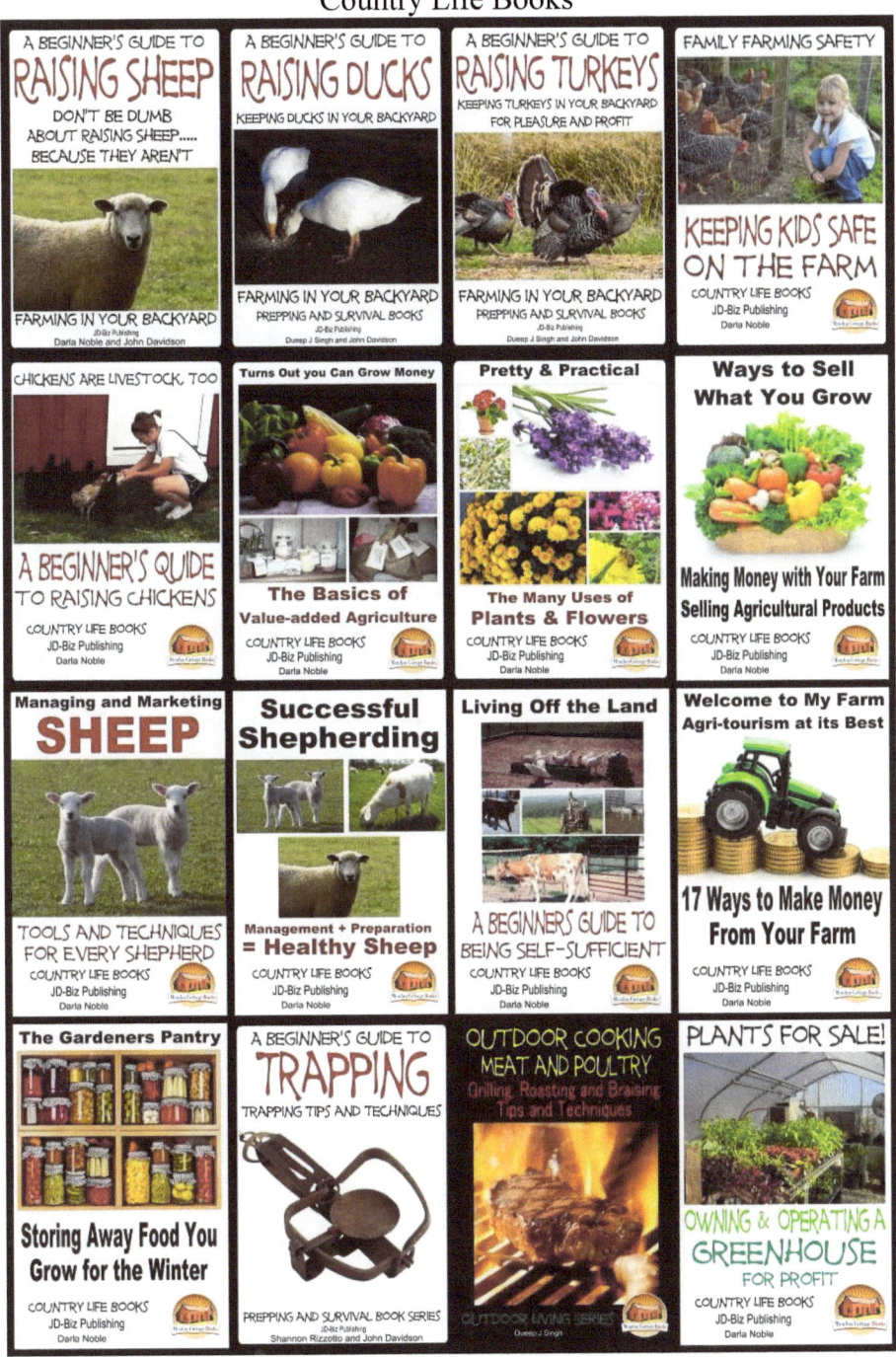

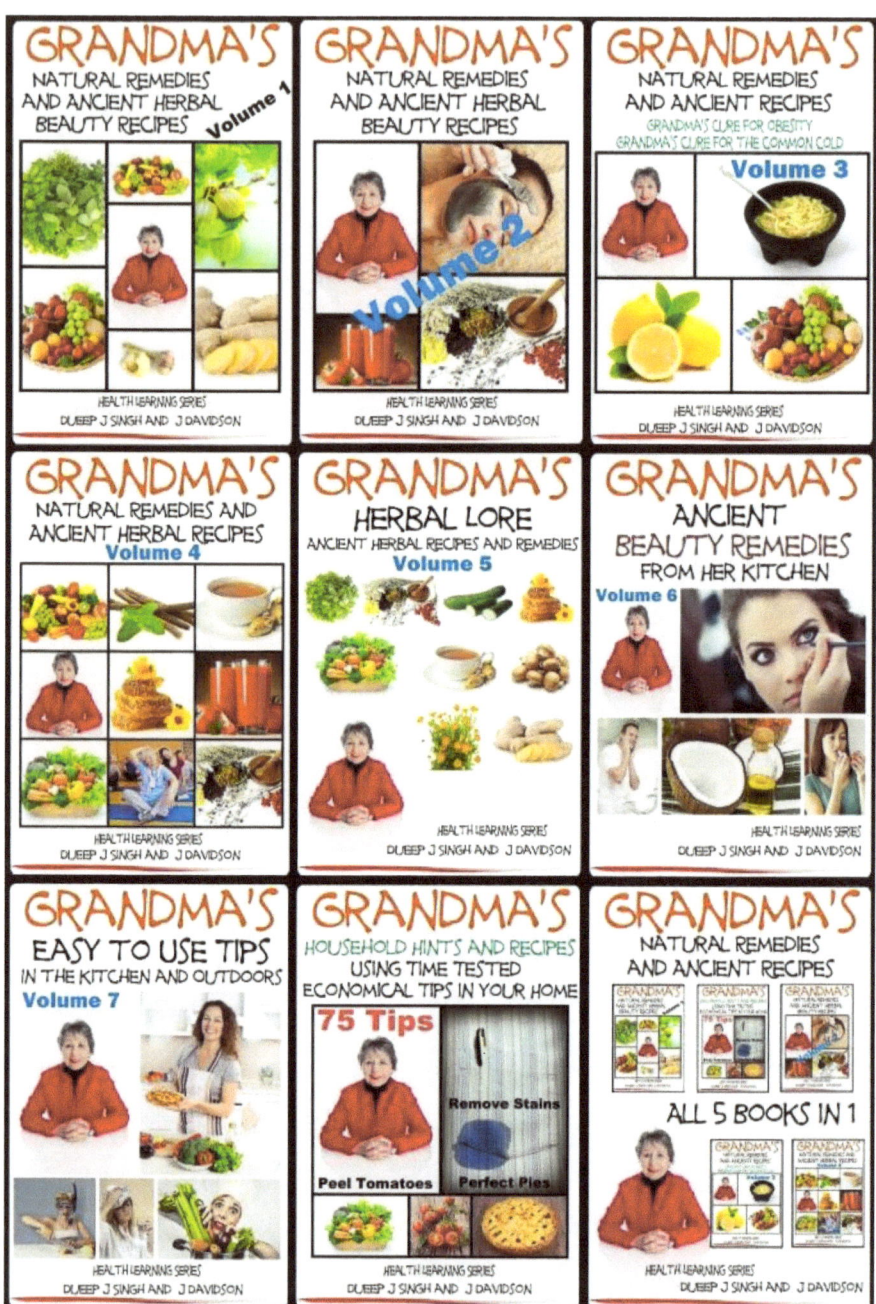

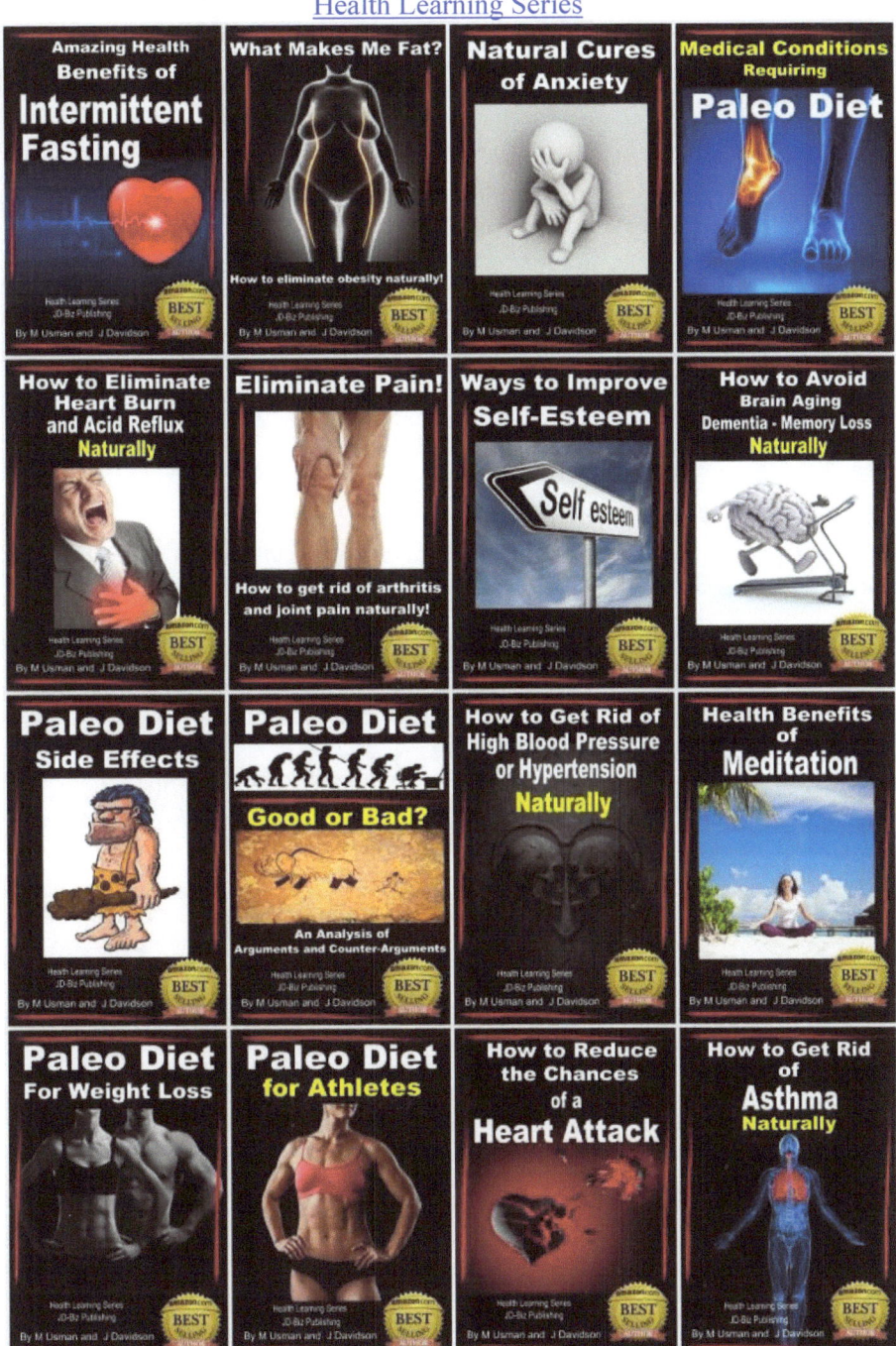

Amazing Animal Book Series

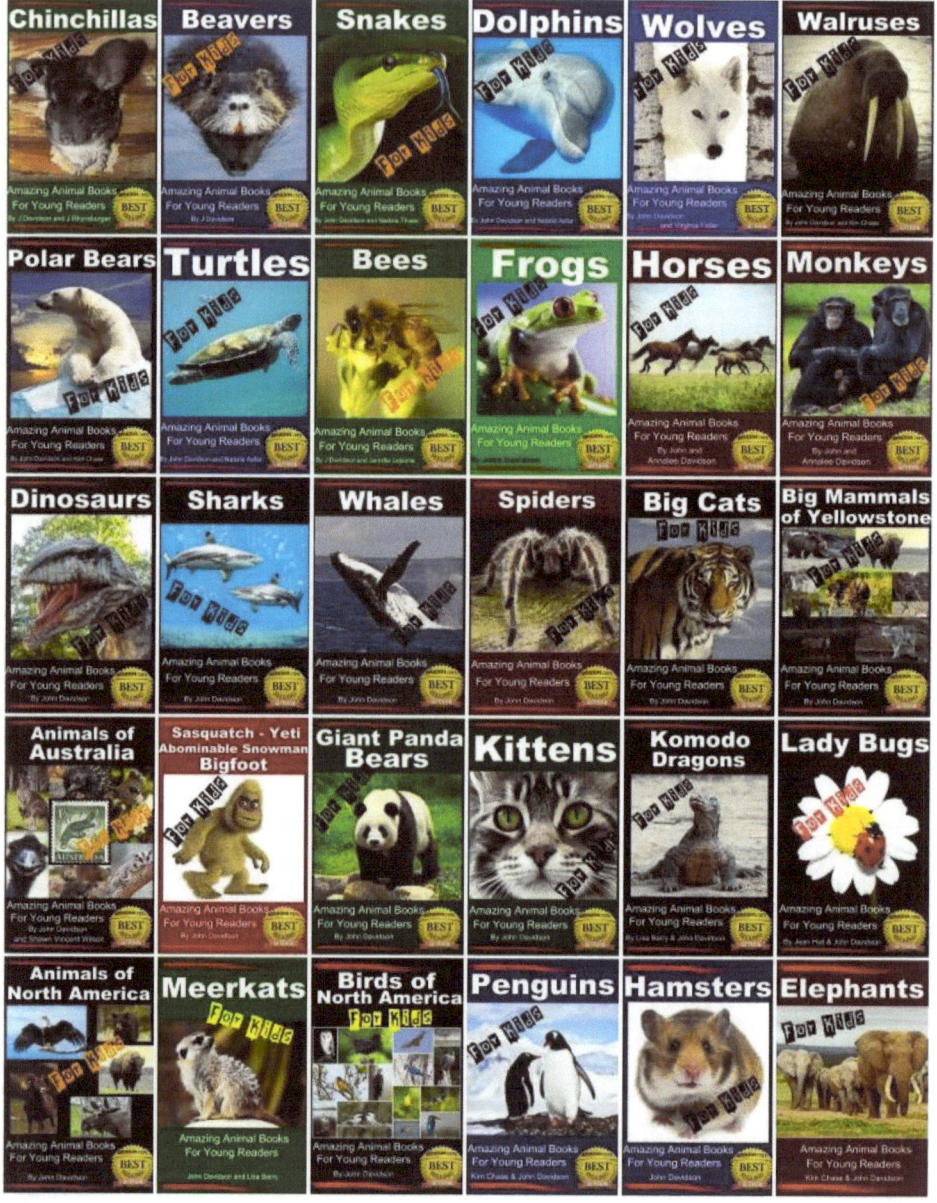

Learn To Draw Series

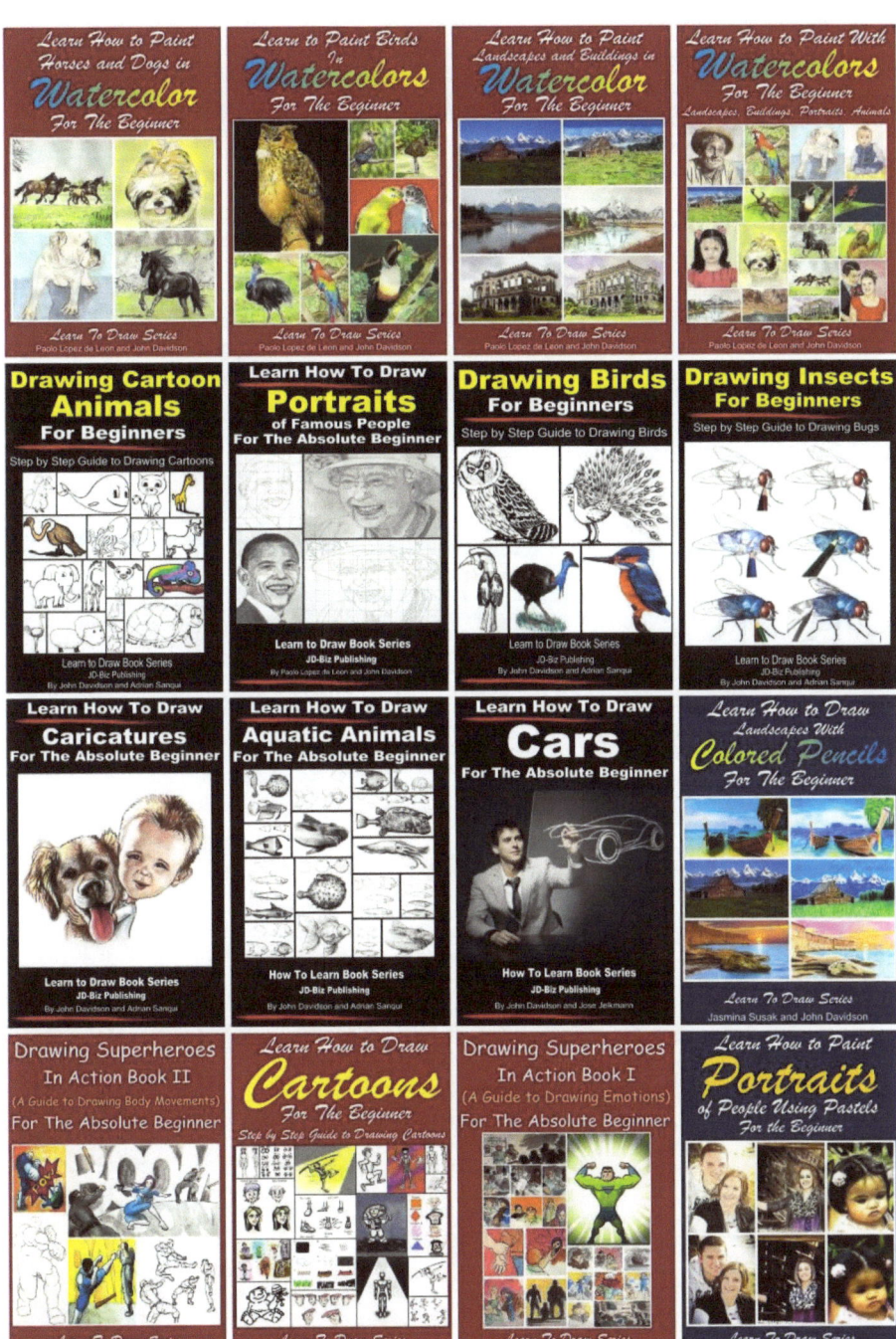

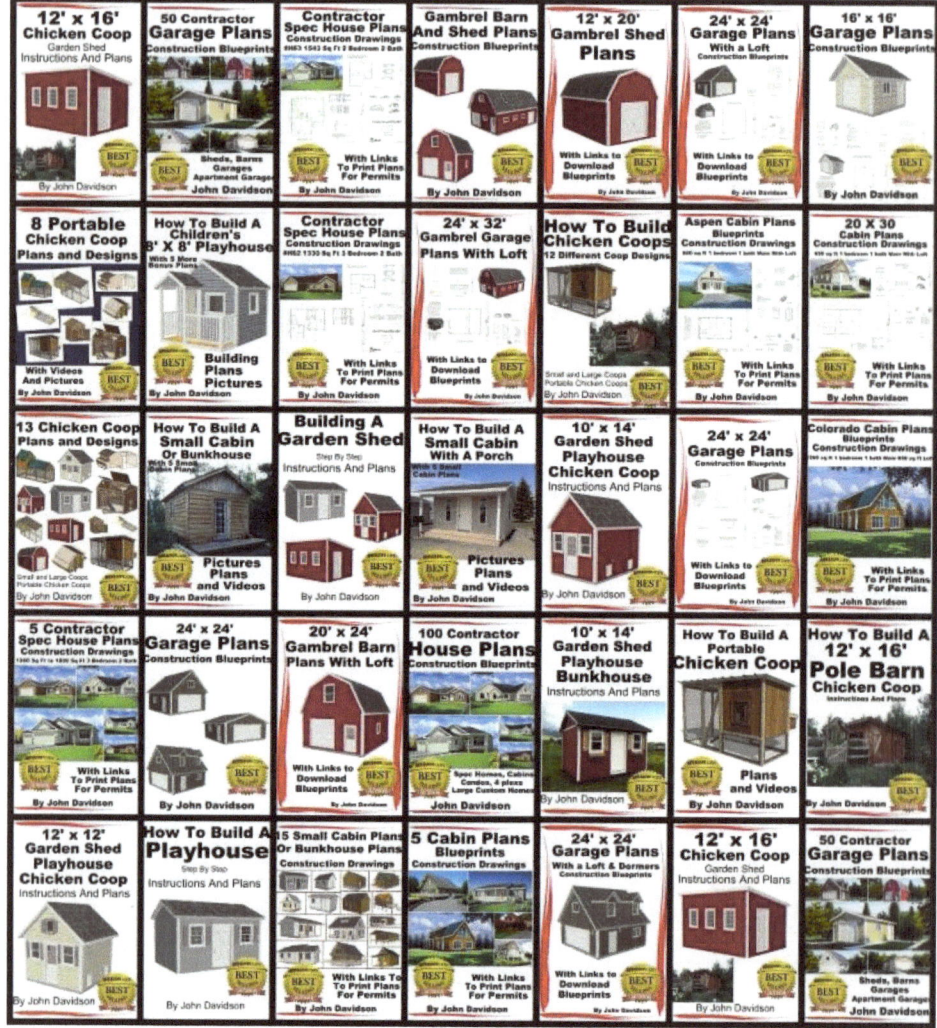

Entrepreneur Book Series

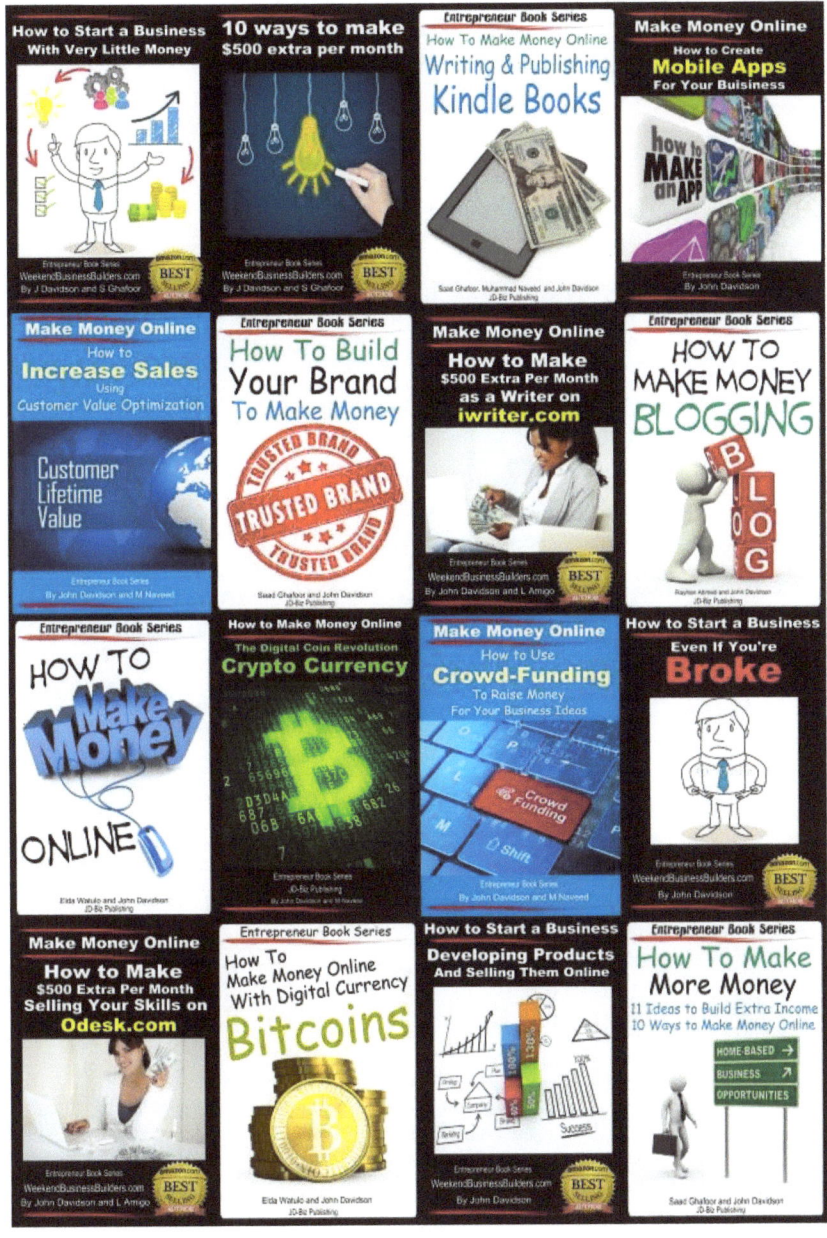

Our books are available at

1. Amazon.com

2. Barnes and Noble

3. Itunes

4. Kobo

5. Smashwords

6. Google Play Books

Download Free Books!

http://MendonCottageBooks.com

Publisher

JD-BIZ PUBLISHING

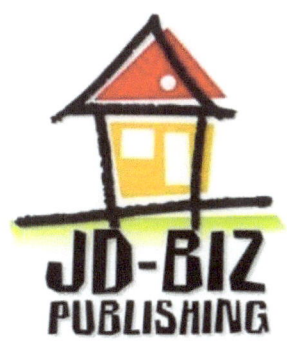

JD-Biz Corp

P O Box 374

Mendon, Utah 84325

http://www.jd-biz.com/

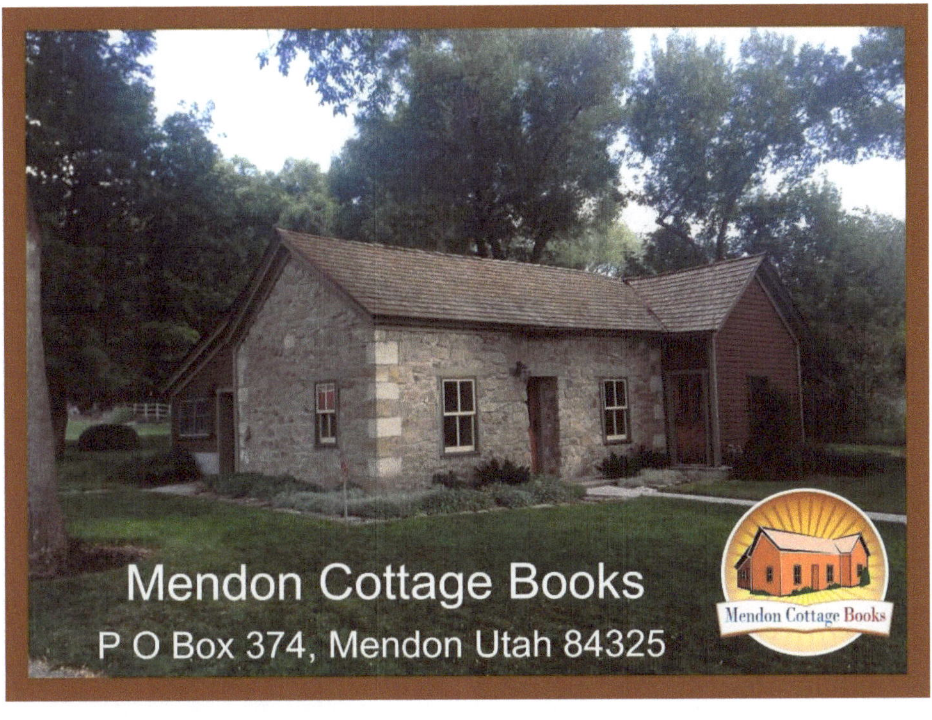

Mendon Cottage Books
P O Box 374, Mendon Utah 84325
Mendon Cottage Books